A PRACTICAL GUIDE
TO HELPING CHILDREN
WITH
SPEECH AND LANGUAGE
PROBLEMS

A PRACTICAL GUIDE
TO HELPING CHILDREN
WITH
SPEECH AND LANGUAGE
PROBLEMS

For Parents and Teachers Only

By

CAROL G. ROUSEY, Ph.D.

Consultant to Preschool Programs
Topeka, Kansas

With Forewords by

Lucile M. Ware, M.D.

Landace Logan Groves

and

Theresa Counts

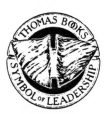

CHARLES C THOMAS • PUBLISHER
Springfield • Illinois • U.S.A.

Published and Distributed Throughout the World by
CHARLES C THOMAS • PUBLISHER
2600 South First Street
Springfield, Illinois 62717

© *1984 by* CHARLES C THOMAS • PUBLISHER

ISBN 0-398-04947-5

Library of Congress Catalog Card Number: 83-18308

With THOMAS BOOKS *careful attention is given to all details of manufacturing and
design. It is the Publisher's desire to present books that are satisfactory as to their physical
qualities and artistic possibilities and appropriate for their particular use.* THOMAS
BOOKS *will be true to those laws of quality that assure a good name and good will.*

Printed in the United States of America
Q-R-3

Library of Congress Cataloging in Publication Data
Rousey, Carol G.
    A practical guide to helping children with speech and
language problems.

    Bibliography: p.
    Includes index.
    1. Speech therapy. 2. Speech disorders in children.
I. Title.
LB3454.R67   1984   371.91'4   83-18308
ISBN 0-398-04947-5

FOREWORD

HERE I have a chance to speak my mind! But what if I couldn't very well, or what if people couldn't understand me? What if I couldn't let my neighbor know I wanted to be friends? How could I tell the teacher what I know or think in class?

Parents and teachers quite reasonably want their children to use speech and language fluently. They become appropriately concerned when something seems amiss. Dr. Carol Rousey now provides parents and teachers with succinct answers to these important questions about speech and language.

This is an impressive volume for its sophistication and its down-to-earth style. While this book can be read at a single sitting, it will merit being reread and studied in depth by parents and teachers concerned about a child with a speech or language problem.

It has been my good fortune as a child psychiatrist to have spent much of my professional career working with the very young child — the child under six. I am only too well aware of

1. the tremendous complexity of growth and development that needs to take place during the earliest formative years
2. the frequency of stresses and strains that impinge

v

upon this growing child (A very, very partial list of stresses would include birth of siblings, moves, illness, separations, divorce, poverty, violence, and so forth.)

3. the many dedicated, caring adults who care for young children at home, in centers, and in schools and who are often overworked and underpaid

4. the relative dearth of support services available for parents and teachers to turn to when there are questions and concerns.

Dr. Rousey makes it clear that speech and language problems merit the urgent concern of the adults around the young child. She describes how and why speech substitutions and distortions should be red flags and alert us that all is not well. She argues cogently for a thoughtful look at the whole child. She presents a systematic way of going about this for the parent or teacher.

Thus, parent or teacher (or both together) can then, once their assessment has been made, follow the prescriptions that Dr. Rousey has so clearly set forth. These guidelines, if thoughtfully studied and carefully applied, I believe, can go a long way toward moving a child out of potential danger and towards a more comfortable developmental path.

Lucile M. Ware, M.D.
Director, Preschool Day Treatment Center
The Menninger Foundation —
Children's Division
Topeka, Kansas

FOREWORD

A TITLE is limited in its ability to describe effectively the material it represents. Dr. Rousey's book is no exception. If her title could truly be descriptive of the information within, it would contain such phrases as "for preservice teachers," "an *essential* guide," "for helping children through the normal stressful situations of childhood," and more!

As a teacher-educator, I highly applaud her research and recommendations supporting the holistic approach to speech and language development. Too often we forget the whole child and focus on only one aspect of growth or learning. Dr. Rousey reminds us that social and emotional developmental needs must be met in order to alleviate speech and language problems.

This book is extremely useful to preservice and inservice teachers as well as parents and others who work closely with young children. In her book, Dr. Rousey briefly gives essential background information about speech and language in easily understood terminology. Then she reviews normal development and identifies potential problem areas through examples. As she relates the two, her suggestions for helping children cope with normal development situations become prescriptions for correcting speech and language problems.

As one who has repeatedly invited Dr. Rousey to share her expertise with university early childhood education classes, I'm grateful now to have access to this unique approach to speech and language problems through this practical guide!

Landace Logan Groves
Early Childhood Education
College of Education
Emporia State University
Emporia, Kansas

FOREWORD

THIS book is not designed as a textbook but rather as a handy reference for parents and teachers. It answers many questions commonly asked by those persons who work or live with children.

A Practical Guide to Helping Children with Speech and Language Problems explains in understandable terms the differing theories of speech therapy — developmental speech therapy versus traditional speech therapy. It also explains why it is important for the whole child to be considered when trying to determine the extent of his difficulty.

The suggestions given make this a very useable tool for both parents and teachers.

At last, a book that answers questions about some of the real speech concerns!

Theresa Counts
Director, Head Start Program
Topeka, Kansas

ACKNOWLEDGMENTS

THE concept of developmental speech therapy has been the culmination of ideas originally advanced through the work of Clyde L. Rousey, Ph.D., and his contribution to the completion of this book is gratefully acknowledged. He has been both my teacher and my husband, a rare combination. In addition, I am sincerely appreciative of all the children, parents, and teachers who have been the living examples of the relevance and usefulness of the ideas expressed in this book. Since practical experience is often the most meaningful, this book is dedicated to my own children, Wayne and Steven.

CONTENTS

A PRACTICAL GUIDE
TO HELPING CHILDREN
WITH
SPEECH AND LANGUAGE
PROBLEMS

Chapter I

INTRODUCTION

THIS book is being written to present a workable, practical guide to helping children who have difficulty in verbal communication. These difficulties may take many forms, such as general delay in development, speech that is hard to understand, or difficulty with specific sound production. This can be a very frustrating experience both on the part of the child who feels unhappy or embarrassed that people cannot understand his attempts at communication and on the part of the adult who is earnestly trying to determine what the child wants or needs.

Issues discussed in this book are addressed specifically to parents and preschool teachers because they are the two groups of people who initially are faced with decisions about a child's communication. Quite often adults will not know if a child has a real problem or if it is only transitory, which leads to decisions about whether or not to obtain specific help, such as from a speech pathologist. Also, when there is an interference with communication, other questions are raised, such as intelligence or broader developmental questions. It is difficult for parents and teachers to understand why one particular child has a great deal of difficulty in verbal communication and another child of the same chronological age (or siblings) seems to have no difficulty whatsoever. In these days of preschools, day care, and increased mobility of families, parents and teachers are exposed to large numbers of children, which leads to comparisons in all phases of development, such as ability to walk, run, climb, and talk. Therefore, concerns are more commonly raised nowadays as levels of expectations of preschoolers are raised.

There are many common questions that occur concerning communication problems. Some of the most often expressed are "Will the child outgrow the problem?" "Is there a physical cause for the problem?" "Why can the child make the sounds correctly sometimes and not at others? Does this mean he's just being stubborn?" Of course, there is no one easy answer to all these questions, but we will try to give some guidelines for making decisions about each child that may be having difficulty.

General Concepts Behind Developmental Speech and Language

The concepts discussed in this section will be termed *developmental* to differentiate them from the traditional methods of therapy discussed in the next section. The developmental method of looking at speech problems has been an outgrowth of the author's experience with traditional methods of therapy and realizing the need to expand our way of thinking to determine how speech and language can fit into the picture of the *whole child* in terms of mental, emotional, and physical growth and development. Too often relationships among all of these areas are not interwoven into a comprehensive view of total development. Different disciplines involved in helping children are not often enough coordinated in their attempts at helping children. The physical needs get taken care of by one person, nutritional needs by another, educational by a third. Under the best of circumstances, all of the areas of a child's development program will provide a consistent program of meeting the needs of each individual in the most efficient, helpful manner. That is why developmental speech therapy takes into account a child's physical, cognitive, and emotional development as an integral part of speech and language development. Therefore, any difficulty in one of these areas should affect other areas, if we can assume that a child develops as a cooordinated whole and not in specific separated parts. This concept is quite often discussed, but when it comes to actually dealing on a day-to-day basis with the child, specific areas are "staked out" by different disciplines and dealt with as if each particular part would be amenable to therapy without directly affecting the others.

Developmental methods of speech therapy have been found useful in both screening and therapy procedures with more than 1,000 children from a wide variety of racial, ethnic, socioeconomic, intellectual, and emotional levels. The factors and concepts discussed apply equally and without bias to all children. There are no specific articulation errors or language misuses that unequivocally differentiate the above noted levels. Granted, there may be culturally accepted methods of expression that are learned by the child that are more readily accepted within certain social situations, but these are beyond the scope of the discussion of developmental learning of speech sounds and language.

Traditional Therapy Methods

A word of explanation should be given about what is traditionally thought of as speech therapy. This method has been generally concerned with exercises and ear training that are outside of the experience of general learning of speech and language skills. Given no undue experiences or limitations, we all learn to talk without any particular drill or attention paid to how we pronounce words, hold our mouth or tongue, or hear the differences between the *right* and *wrong* way to say sounds or words. When a child is enrolled in traditional speech therapy in most clinical or school settings today, there is a sequence that is most generally followed that includes ear training to learn the differences between correct and incorrect sound production, visual and tactile assistance in correct placement of lips and tongue, and various drills to incorporate consistent use of the sound in words and sentences and then finally into usage in everyday conversation. The general assumption is that sounds are either mislearned or not learned for unknown reasons, and proper teaching methods and consequent rewards will motivate the child toward correct sound or language use. Little attention is directed to learning the *why* of misarticulation or misuse of language, but a great deal of attention is given to *what* is incorrect. Traditional methods of therapy assume a learning or cognitive basis with motivation for change being, at least initially, largely supplied by the clinician or therapist. Motivational techniques include rewarding the child with points, stickers, verbal praise, winning of speech games, or edibles. All this is done so that the child will form correct habits of sound or language production. Despite the fact that we learn to talk by listening to and interacting with other individuals in our environment with all the attendant interpersonal forces coming into play, traditional speech therapy is done in a structured learning situation in a classroom or office.

Differences Between Speech and Language

We will discuss speech and language as two separate entities, but closely linked in the general development of a child. Speech will refer to the individual sounds of our language, i.e., /r/, /s/, /v/. On the surface they carry out no overt meaning by themselves and are called *phonemes* in the language of speech pathologists. When sounds are put together into meaningful units that constitute communicative messages, we have language. For instance, the word *me* would be made up of two separate phonemes, /m/ and /e/, but when put together make up the pronoun *me*. Individually, sounds are meaningless and are made from birth but only become incorporated into a language system at about one year of age.

It is important to keep the difference between speech and language in mind when we talk about development. Quite often the terms are used interchangeably, but for the purposes of this book we will differentiate between the two concepts. This is done because speech and language involve different aspects of development and carry entirely different meanings when we talk about levels of development.

Red Flag Approach

When we think of how speech (individual sounds) or language (sounds put together into words) develop in children, we realize that no particular drill or teaching methods are used. Children learn to speak generally because they are spoken to by adults and other children in their environment, and they learn to communicate with others because they hear other people talk. We do not receive any formal classes in learning to say the word *table* or *mama* or *dog*, for we just hear other people use these words meaningfully and then incorporate them into our own way of communicating our needs and feelings to other people. The question then arises about why sometimes problems occur with the saying of particular words or sounds. When a child starts out saying the word /tat/ instead of /cat/, we wonder why it is that the child is misarticulating the initial sound of the word but not why the rest of the word is said correctly. Chances are that the child has not heard anyone say the word /tat/ instead of /cat/. Another example might be a child who has trouble using the pronoun /me/ in place of /I/, such as when saying the sentence "Me want that." Children do not start out hearing adults using pronouns this way. Therefore, we can conclude that learning of correct sound usage and pronoun usage does not come from the environment or other people but must be determined by some factor other than can be explained by a simple learning process.

These rules of grammar that we all learn just by listening to other people talk usually go unanalyzed by most of us. Although we are not aware of specific grammar rules as we talk with each other, we do know that sentences are put together in a certain way with certain parts of speech. Children talk in fairly complex sentences by the age of five, although if they had to diagram or identify parts of verbal language, they would be unable to do so. This applies not only to children but also to adults, unless we are sitting in an English grammar classroom. However, we all skillfully speak so that we can be understood by others and do a pretty good job of putting nouns, pronouns, and verbs in the proper sequence. Therefore, *grammar*, as in the case of *sounds*, is *learned* through practice in verbal communication with others. This lends support to the idea that we do not mislearn sounds or words because we have not heard them misused by others in our environment.

Carrying this concept a step further, we can then begin to think that any deviation from the general developmental learning process can be considered a red flag and allow ourselves to investigate the *why* of the misarticulation or misuse of pronouns. The ideas developed in this book will address this concept of a red flag and consider that speech or language difficulties are warning signals that a child is having some extra amount of difficulty with a particular stage of normal development and could benefit from special attention from parents, teachers, or other interested adults. If we recognize the red flag, then a closer more critical look at the child will help us determine what seems to be of particular concern, either by viewing the behavior patterns during the course of daily routine or by scheduling an evaluation from an appropriately trained professional. Instead of just focusing on the speech or language of a child and treating these areas in isolation from the whole individual, we can direct our concern to what the child is trying to tell us with his red flag and why he needs to have some additional attention paid to certain developmental needs.

Myths Concerned with Speech and Language

Having laid our original assumptions concerning speech and language development and the red flag approach to difficulties, we can now begin to look at some new answers to the questions raised at the beginning of this chapter.

1. *Will the child outgrow this problem?* Quite often parents and teachers do not become concerned with any difficulties that preschoolers may have with speech, because as adults it seems that we have all more or less outgrown any specific sound or language difficulties. However, this attitude does not take notice of the issue implied in the manifestation of the problem. Because the speech/language difficulty occurs, it means that there is a specific need in development that has occurred and is important to the child. If the concerned adult is truly interested in helping the child make the best possible adjustment in development, then the issue of "waiting to outgrow" the need becomes of secondary importance. The adult will be most concerned with what he can do *at the time* to help the child in making an easier adjustment to current concerns.

2. *Is there a physical cause for the problem?* This should be first of all a question ruled out by the family physician or child's pediatrician. If no overt cause is present, such as a cleft palate or hearing impairment, then further attention should be paid to general developmental needs of the child. With a few exceptions, such as the two just cited, there are no direct relationships between speech and language impairments and physical manifestations.

3. *Why can the child make sounds correctly sometimes and not at others?* This particular situation indicates there is no physical cause for misarticulation. Therefore, there must be other determining factors present and paying careful attention to these issues will assist the child in speeding up and finalizing correct sound usage.

4. *Has the child picked up bad speaking habits from others?* A yes answer to this question would have to assume that

there is only one speech model present for the child, i.e., the family member or other individual with the speech problem. In all practicality this is very unlikely. There are many speech models present in the lives of most children, and it would seem very difficult for a child to only listen to one person with a speech difficulty and to imitate their speech directly in the face of all the other models present.

5. *Should we drill the child on the sounds that are difficult?* I always ask the parents who have done this if the exercise has been successful, and the overwhelming answer is, "No, it just seems to make it worse," or "My child just ignores me." These situations occur because the speech sounds are not based on cognitive learning principles but are stemming from deeper developmental needs that are not under the direct conscious control of the child. As a rule of thumb, it should always be assumed that children are talking or expressing themselves to the very best of their ability and are only limited by noncognitive developmental issues.

Summary

In this introductory chapter we have presented a brief explanation of the differences between traditional developmental speech and language concepts. A rationale for using the broader more encompassing concept of developmental theory has been presented using the red flag approach as a basis for recognizing these needs.

Chapter II
EARLY STAGES OF DEVELOPMENT

A S stated in the introductory chapter, the type of speech and language we will be concerned with is directly related to developmental stages in a child's life. Therefore, this chapter will present an overview of generally recognized levels so that we can see how the whole child develops and relate some concerns about special helps that may be needed at each of these times. Material has been drawn from different disciplines and theoretical viewpoints (Doll, 1965; Engle, 1963; Frankenburg and Dodds, 1969; Knoblock and Pasamanick, 1974; Zimmerman, Steiner, and Evatt, 1969).

The material will be presented chronologically to facilitate discussion, although it must be remembered that there is a wide variance among children, and it may be impossible to determine exactly at what stage a particular child may be in terms of fitting neatly into the categories presented. Also, there may be overlapping areas. However, the stages of development can be used as a general outline to assess levels of functioning or to assist in pinpointing areas of particular difficulty.

Our discussion will relate physical and psychological stages so that the relationship between the two can be seen and then directly related to speech and language development. Material presented from the several authors is characteristic of a wealth of information that can be found in many different sources. It is hoped that this summary will be a concise, representative sample of child development. The chart on the next page presents the information in outline form.

The First Year (Zero to Twelve Months)

Dramatic changes are made both physically, socially, and psychologically during this first year of life. A baby progresses from confinement in a stationary position to being able to roll over, crawl, and stand alone to perhaps taking a few steps alone. In addition, the child can reach and grasp desired objects. There should also be some ability to follow simple instructions, such as waving goodbye.

At the same time these physical changes are occurring, there are specific emotional needs that are required to insure a solid basis of confidence in the child's world. These needs center around a sureness of getting nurturance, both in actual feeding activities and in a physical and emotional loving. If this feeling of love and trust is incorporated early in life, then the child will feel comfortable in separating briefly from loved ones, confident that they will be there upon return. Also during the first year the child will form the basis of moving from a completely self-centered world into the concept of being a separate individual who lives in communication with other people. This awareness will require some adaption on his part. Initially, the baby will feel a sameness with the mother. During this time, he regards himself as the center and

	SPEECH and LANGUAGE	PHYSICAL	SOCIAL/PSYCHOLOGICAL/COGNITIVE
1st Year C.A. 0-12 months	Undifferentiated vocalizations Ability to understand simple words Says first word	Reaches and grasps Rolls over Crawls Stands alone Follows simple instructions	Requires sureness of nurturant needs (food, loving) Self-centered world Learns self-differentiation from others Learning to separate and return to trusted others
2nd Year C.A. 1-2 years	Vocabulary of 50-100 words Uses two words together in speaking Beginning to develop grammar	True walking, running Help with simple self-care Single and cooperative play Fetches or carries familiar objects Goes about house or yard	Awareness of people and things and ability to remember them Pleasure in self-accomplishment Curiosity about body parts Learning to conform to or defy parental standards
3rd Year C.A. 2-3 years	Great vocabulary growth Pleasure in talking to others Uses three words together in speaking	Refinement of motor skills, i.e., uses eating utensils, cuts with scissors, dries own hands Remove coat or dress Gets drink unassisted Avoids simple hazards	Learns social and sexual differences Continues to refine conflict between satisfying own needs and conforming to standards Learning physical and verbal limits
4th Year C.A. 3-4 years	Uses four words together in speaking Using conjunctions and prepositions	Can skip on one foot Copy a cross Help with small household tasks Walks down stairs one step per tread Buttons Washes hands unaided	Continued modification of personal drive wishes Growing self-confidence in social acceptance Emerging intact superego
5th Year C.A. 4-5 years	Uses five words together in speaking— similar to adults Uses most sentence forms Uses "why" questions	Cares for self in toileting Dresses self except for tying Uses pencil or crayon for drawing Can balance and hop on one foot Catches a ball	Comprehends prepositions Enjoys competitive exercise games Confidence in going about neighborhood unattended Can verbally relate solutions to problems of being sleepy, hungry, cold Knows concept of opposites

most important thing and assumes that the world only consists of a means to get demands satisfied. However, an awareness should grow on the part of the infant that he is separate and differentiated from the mother.

This first year, then, contains several distinct developmental stages that are either met or left uncompleted. We can briefly identify them as (1) a sense of nurturance, both physically and emotionally, (2) development of a sense of trust in other individuals with regard to the sureness of this nurturance, and (3) ability to separate successfully and return to these trusted individuals.

The Second Year (One to Two Years of Age)

During the months between one and two years of age, a child makes rapid progress in the development of motor skills that will include mastery of walking and running as well as the ability to assist with simple self-care activities such as dressing. During this time there is also a developing ability to discriminate edible from nonedible substances. Specific play activities will start to be initiated by the child in addition to some cooperative play with others. As a part of his increased mobility and socialization, the child develops an increasing confidence in going about and exploring the house and outside yard alone without needing quite so quickly to return to the parent. This confidence is enhanced if the appropriate trusting feelings have been successfully mastered.

Psychologically, the child continues to develop the awareness of his own separate identity apart from other individuals and to learn that people and objects can be mentally represented or remembered when out of sight. It has been theorized that this may be the beginning of true intelligent behavior. A child may think of himself in relation to other individuals and objects in his environment and begin to speculate about his own identity and role in these relationships. It may be at this point that the concept of cause and effect is first established.

During this year there is also a developing pleasure in self-accomplishment but at the same time a concern over the possible dangers that may be present. This is a transitional stage between venturing out on his own and relying on the adults in the world for assistance. There is a delicate balance between allowing a child to develop at his own self-regulated pace and either holding back or pushing him too fast.

This second year is when a child is asked to start to learn to conform to adult wishes in certain socially acceptable areas. Because of newly developed feelings of independence, a child feels he has a choice now of either conforming to or defying these adult wishes. There can be an air of easy cooperation and learning to share during this period, or a child may feel he can successfully demonstrate control over his own body in defiance of what parents want. One area that often is picked as a battleground over these rights is that of toileting. For the first time a child may feel he has control over internal bodily functions that are independent of parental influence and may choose to demonstrate or act out his reluctance to cooperate easily in the bathroom. Because there are so many cultural overtones concerning this issue, many parents engage in battle without viewing the issue from the larger perspective of a period during which a child needs to learn how to cooperate and share with others within adult preset standards.

Important stages during this second year may be summarized as (1) learning to conform to or defy standards

set by parents that is characterized by a willingness or difficulty in cooperation, (2) pleasure in self-accomplishment done at the child's appropriate pace, and (3)
growing self-concept and identity.

The Third Year (Two to Three Years of Age)

Physically, between two and three years of age, the
child continues to refine motor skills, i.e., to learn to use
eating utensils and to cut with a pair of scissors. He can
dry his own hands and remove a coat or dress and get a
drink of water unassisted. In addition, there is an increased ability to take care of himself and to avoid simple
hazards.

This year is the start of primary social and sexual dif-
ferentiation when a child learns that there are important
and real differences between being a male or a female.
This brings up the necessity for identification with a particular sex model and an awareness of how this identification contrasts with the opposite sex. There may be noted
differences in how the child behaves toward the mother as
opposed to the father in the family. Children need two
role models (male and female) to observe and contrast so
that they can clearly see and differentiate how adults of
both sexes act, talk, look, feel, and sound.

Continuing the earlier process of conforming to or defying adult authority, a child is learning the limits of satisfying his own needs while still fitting in comfortably with
what parents and other adults expect or demand. These
adult figures must provide a firm, reassuring outer
boundary within which a child can mold his own needs
and desires. These limits can be both physical and verbal.
Real opportunities for social self-control are present when
a child is confronted with a strong desire or need, which

must be modified into socially (parental) acceptable means of expression.

There should be a good healthy exploration of how far physical and verbal limits can be tested safely with the secure knowledge that boundaries will remain constant and firm. These limits will need to be outlined again and again until the child internalizes them and they become part of his own thoughts. Physical boundaries (such as not going out into the street) are often more obvious than verbal because they may involve factors of safety for the child. However, all children need to learn appropriate verbal assertiveness to hold their own in social interactions. This is in contrast to a tough and aggressive way of dealing with people that results in a demanding, order giving, bossy sort of verbal behavior.

Important stages that are dealt with through this third year may be summarized as (1) primary social and sexual identification with role models being important and (2) learning how to appropriately interact within physical and verbal limits.

The Fourth Year (Three to Four Years of Age)

A child between the ages of three and four is learning how to engage in true cooperative play and can enjoy performing for others. Motor coordination has improved to the point where it is possible to skip on one foot, button clothing, and walk down stairs one step per tread. There should also be developing some ability to help at small tasks around the home.

Psychologically, there is a continued modification of ways a child uses to satisfy his needs within the bounds of environmental demands. Since these modifications become increasingly socially acceptable, they result in a growing self-confidence of social acceptance. An emerging sense of identity and self-concept allows the child to interact in the world away from constant supervision by parental figures. Real strides are made in combining all these factors in an effort to consolidate the unique individuality of the child.

This year can be summarized as being important in continuing the growth both physically and psychologically, work that has ideally had a solid basis for easy growth and development as the child matures.

The Fifth Year (Four to Five Years of Age)

Physically a child can now dress himself with some assistance in areas such as tying and can care for himself in toileting. Motor skills have developed so that a pencil or crayon can be used for drawing. At this age a child may also be able to balance on one foot, hop, and even catch a ball.

Socially and cognitively there is now an enjoyment of competitive exercise games with other children and a confidence in going about the immediate neighborhood unattended by a parent. Cognitively, a child should be starting to comprehend the concept of opposites, such as big versus little, and to understand the idea of prepositions, such as up, down, and over. Verbally, there is some ability to relate solutions to daily problems such as being cold, sleepy, or hungry.

In summary, the child between the ages of four and five continues to build on and consolidate the physical, social, and cognitive growth of previous years. There is a continued push toward self-awareness and confidence in one's own capabilities and skill in dealing with the environment and figures in it.

Summary

Chapter II has presented a brief overview of general stages of development in the areas of physical, social/ psychological growth. We have seen the child go from a dependent infant to an independent individual who ideally is free to separate from caring adults, share with others, and modify personal needs within the framework of societal standards.

Chapter III
HOW COMMUNICATION THROUGH LANGUAGE DEVELOPS

General Concepts

It will be remembered that in an earlier chapter we discussed the difference between language and speech sounds. Language, to be consistent, will be thought of in this chapter to consist of the stringing together of sounds to form a system of verbal communication, while speech is assumed to refer to the individual sounds within this system. The individual sounds within our language will be discussed in the following chapter.

Although language can take many forms such as gestures, writing, and sign language, we will discuss communication through verbal language in this chapter. This part of communication is a specific function of the human species that allows us to map our experiences through spoken words. This idea suggests that humans are *prewired* to use verbal language. When a child is learning a specific language, the task then becomes how to apply a set of innate abstract rules to make language work in a particular cultural environment. This issue may speak to the critical place of feedback from others in the child's environment that allows a youngster to try out a particular set of sounds or combination of sounds to determine how language can be useful in development. Lenneberg (1967) has supported the concept of an inborn language capacity because there does not seem to be any evidence that language emerges as a response to an external need or utility initially. There is also the phenomenon that language development follows the same general sequence from the utterance of the first word throughout all cultures, but we usually are unaware of these rules unless specifically taught.

Once the individual responds to this innate need to develop language, there is the beginning of a communication system through use of the sounds and then words of a language. The *magic* properties of language are discussed by Fraiberg (1959). She suggests that language originates in a *magic* type of setting. For example, the use of sounds can *magically* make a mother or other caretaker appear from out of eyesight. Later a child learns that the word *mama* (or other word approximating caring adults) can bring great excitement and pleasure in reciprocation. In addition, if this same word is thought about silently, it can give a permanence and stability to the mental image of the mother, recreate the positive feeling of nurturance, and, therefore, reduce the anxiety of separation. This phenomenon was observed by the author while working with a four-year-old boy who had recently been hospitalized for a few days and then had returned to the therapy setting. He was able to separate easily from his mother for the therapy session but then found himself anxious about leaving her in the adjoining waiting room. He could be heard softly to repeat *mama* to himself several times, smile, and then return to therapy activities. He was being reassured by the simple repetition of the word that to him represented comfort and caring.

In addition, although we are speaking specifically about language of children, it is important to know that all through our lives we use this magic of language. To extend this idea further, not just children, but adults use language to give themselves comfort in times of stress. When we are separated from a loved one, even as an adult, we use internal language to recreate experiences and the image of that individual so that we can be comforted during their absence. We also mentally, in times of stress, rehearse language that we will use. We plan ahead what we will say to a particular individual, or we rehearse internally a speech that we are going to give so that we can feel more psychologically comfortable. Language, then, can be used to reduce stress and tension and make ourselves feel more comfortable or can help ease the pain of loneliness. In a positive sense, we also recreate situations that we have had to make ourselves feel good by reliving a particular event in our life.

Language has served additional functions in the changes humankind has made over the span of the centuries. One useful function of language has been its survival value. From the earliest development of a communication system, language has been important in helping man survive the dangers in the environment. We have managed to survive more easily and efficiently by being able to warn others of imminent danger through language. This idea can be applied from the earliest language of the caveman to current times when parents warn their children to be careful crossing the street or not to poke their fingers in light sockets.

Another function of language is that it can be used to result in behavioral changes and allows man to modify the environment around him. Children apply this concept by voicing likes and dislikes about the things around them. For example, they can tell you if the bath water is too hot or if the food is too cold. Language lets children know they can have an active part in getting assistance to make their lives better or easier.

Language also enables man to go far beyond the bounds of his physical capabilities and experiences. We can watch a documentary on television about a faraway country or read a book that allows us to experience what it would be like to ride on top of an elephant or to go down in a coal mine. These are experiences that most of us will probably never have in real life, but by reading the words or having someone describe it to us, we can recreate the experience for ourselves. This is, of course, one of the reasons why we do so much reading of books to children. It allows them to go on and know what various parts of the world or various experiences are like in the place of or before they actually happen. Thus, age-old human experience can be passed on to children by adults and can assist them in mastering experience and acquiring new modes of behavior.

A child's mental activities are conditioned from an early age by the social relationships with significant adults in their lives. By these social relationships with other adults, children learn appropriate ways of interacting with others. Adults spend a great deal of time, especially with young children, giving them instructions on how to behave. This includes such diverse issues as manners, taking turns, asking for what you want, respecting elders, or saying please and thank you. Children learn that language is a useful tool in getting along with others. It is important that adults realize that children's experiences with verbal language, either negative or positive, come from what they learn from their interactions with adults or from observation of how adults talk with each other.

Language is important, also, in developing an individual's self-concept. We can use language as a medium to put ourselves in the place of someone else and thus help differentiate ourselves from others. It can be used to represent oneself in imaginary situations or play, which assists in identification. We can often overhear young children playing *mommy* or *daddy* or *doctor* or *bus driver*.

Language can be used to internalize standards of our society because a great deal of discussion and direction giving with regard to behavior is done by adults to children, which is then assimilated by the child to monitor behavior. An example to illustrate this concept happened with a four-year-old boy enrolled in a preschool program who was having a great deal of difficulty in controlling his behavior. His teacher, responding to his need for external control, would appropriately remind him that either he could do the requested task or she would help him to do it. After a time, he could be overheard to remind himself verbally, "I can either do it myself, or she'll come and help me do it." Thus, he was able to take the external behavior control of an adult and transfer it to himself and then later internalize it and silently modify his own behavior to correspond to what was expected of him in the classroom.

All of these changes and functions of language hinge on the fact that it has been man who has possessed the physiological brain structure that has been capable of growth and modification over the evolutionary time span. Language is our most useful tool in learning and serves as the most important element in transmittal of information about our past, present, and future growth.

Comprehension versus Performance

In the overall development of language, it is generally assumed that the understanding of a verbal communication system (comprehension) is chronologically ahead of the actual usage (performance) of this system. An example would be when a young child is able to understand a request such as "Bring me the ball" before he can actually speak the entire sentence. Therefore, when discussing a level of ability of a particular child, the difference between understanding and speaking must be kept in mind and any gross discrepancies questioned. A child may adequately understand questions, requests, and directions and yet exhibit almost little or no actual language usage for various reasons. We could say about such a child that his understanding is at a chronologically correct age of four years, but his expressive language is at the eighteen-month level if he is only using approximately one or two words meaningfully. Such differences are important in measuring general developmental levels and in assessing the needs of a particular child.

Factors Affecting Language and Speech (Sound) Acquisition

For purposes of reference, we will divide our discussion of issues that directly affect development of a verbal communication system into four main sections. The first factor is *readiness*. There seems to be a universal preset time for language/speech development. All children the world over manage to acquire communication skills at about the same chronological age — no matter what the language system being learned. There is very little adults can do to speed up this acquisition, to accelerate development, or to encourage particular skill development out of sequence. It is assumed that there is a critical interaction between time and general development that is preprogrammed for communication development. It has also been postulated that if for any reason this critical period is missed, it becomes increasingly difficult for later unencumbered development of communication skills.

The second general area affecting development is that of *physical capacities*. There needs to be certain given physical characteristics that are essential to the development of a workable communication system. These characteristics include an intact auditory system for hearing, intellectual abilities within normal limits, and an absence of any severe neuromuscular or brain-integrating problems. Any one of these problems in the area of physical characteristics can have an important effect on the development of receptive and/or expressive language. These are areas that need to be ruled out by a physical examination, which might include a hearing test by an audiologist who is particularly trained to test the hearing of young children as well as information from the pediatrician.

The third area is that of *environmental influences*. Although the direct cause and effect relationships within this province may be more subjective than objective in nature, nevertheless it is important to recognize the positive or negative effect environmental factors may play. These factors include such diverse areas as (1) child-rearing practices — there may be differences in language development that can be attributed to the child's daily exposure to verbal interactions such as only being in the company of adults, being raised in an institutional setting, or being left in a confined area such as a play pen for long periods of time with little contact with other people and (2) the amount of positive or negative feedback a child receives from his attempts at verbal communication. There may be differences in development due to encouragement or negative reactions to attempts at verbal communication. It is important to know whether the child has been encouraged and smiled upon when first trying to communicate verbally or whether he has been ignored, ridiculed, or told to be quiet. In addition, there should be continuing ample opportunities for language expression. This would include experiences for the child to discuss such as things seen during a walk or participating in verbal exchange during daily activities. One convenient way to examine language interaction between a child and others is to categorize the ways language is used into three main divisions:

   a. Is the child only talked *to* or *at* with no opportunity for participation on the part of the child? This would happen when a child is only told to "Sit down," "Be quiet," "Eat your potatoes," "Put on your coat," "Don't do that again," or "It's time to go now." This type of language can be characterized by a feeling of ordering or commanding that does not expect or want any type of response or discussion from the child.

   b. Is talking done *for* the child so that he need not participate in any way in requesting help or satisfying needs? Parents are sometimes aware that an older brother or sister "interprets" what a younger sibling is saying so that no real need to communicate in an increasingly clear manner exists for the younger child. This also happens when a child becomes used to pointing at desired objects or when every need is anticipated and no choice left up to the child.

c. Is talking done back and forth *with* the child with appropriate ratio of adult and child exchange of information?

We should stress that all of these three areas have their appropriate place in learning to use language. Each type of language should be used in different situations. Our point is that when there is an overwhelming abundance of examples *a* and *b* in a child's life, language development will suffer. These three examples are given as a way to examine the majority of verbal interactions in a child's life.

This third area of environmental influence may or may not be important in its effect on language development. A child's position in the family may make a difference in the amount of time available to both verbally and nonverbally interact with available adults. There may have to be special attention paid to the rights of each family member to have an opportunity to talk on a balanced level with others, no matter what the particular age distribution might be.

The fourth area affecting language acquisition can be thought of as *general criteria* that are necessary in a verbal communication system. Eisenson and Ogilvie (1971) refer to three essential parts of this system. A child may be thought of as having speaking ability when three stages are intact. The first of these is the ability to understand language, which means that the child possesses the means to abstract actual meaning from a preset system of audible or visible symbols. The second stage involves the ability to *listen* creatively and generalize from a past knowledge of this system and then to use this generalization to formulate meanings from new words. The third stage is the ability to *talk* creatively. This means that a child is able to generalize from past utterances to new, previously unspoken combinations of words to generate new speech and verbal experiences. Language development as we will use the term is then essentiallly a two-way street. Its successful use depends upon reception, integration, and expression of a language system through an orderly developmental sequence of generalizations.

How Communication Develops

There are certain generally accepted stages in the development of a communication system, specifically a verbal language, based on chronological norms. Rousey and Rousey (1978) have described these stages in their booklet *Your Child's Speech and Hearing* as follows:

Zero to Twelve months: The development of a child's language is a natural one that starts right after birth. After about two months a baby will make some different sounds when he is happy or hungry. Shortly after this, there may be some specific verbal sound responses to people, and some time before the first birthday there will be echoing of sounds heard from others, although there will probably not be meaning attached to them. During this first year of life babies are known to make all of the sounds contained in our language in a meaningless random fashion, but it should be noted that the physical capabilities of all sound production are present by twelve months.

Twelve months: At about one year of age a child may be starting to understand some simple verbal language, such as when an adult says, "no, no." A child may also be able to follow very simple commands such as, "Wave bye-bye." You will recall we discussed earlier the concept of comprehension preceding production, and this example is a good illustration. The child may be able to wave bye-bye on request and yet be unable actually to produce the spoken word sequence. Thus, he comprehends the meaning of "bye-bye" but is not yet ready to say the words themselves.

Twelve to eighteen months: Between one and two years of age, children's command of language expands rapidly. By eighteen months there should be at least one or two understandable words in a child's vocabulary that are intelligible even to those not familiar with the child. At this age, one word utterances may be thought of as standing for a complete thought, i.e., "Momma" may be uttered in different ways to mean "Where is my mother?" or "Mother, I hurt myself," or "Mommy, I'm glad to see you." He should also be able to recognize some objects from hearing the name of the object spoken, such as when the child is asked to "Show me your ball," he can produce the required object.

Two years: By two years of age, a child's vocabulary has grown from 50 to 100 words, many of which can be understood by others outside the family. He should be using phrases, an average of about two words together at a time, and should be able to follow some verbal directions from others such as "Go find Daddy." At this age, a child is also starting to generate some word combinations that he perhaps has not heard others speak. For instance, he may be saying the phrase "Mommy go" and then altering the next phrase to "Doggy go" so that he is trying out new combinations of words daily. Also during this year most children are starting to use some of what are called functional words, which include conjunctions, articles, and prepositions in their utterance so they may use combinations such as "Sit down, Mommy."

Three years: Between two and three years of age is usually the greatest period of vocabulary growth. A child expands both the number of words and the length of phrases and will demonstrate willingness and pleasure in verbal communication. He may react negatively if others around him have some difficulty understanding his speech. There should be an average of three words in spoken phrases and there may be as many as 1,000 words in the vocabulary.

Four years: By four years of age there is an average length of sentence of four words and spoken language includes conjunctions and prepositions. Language is used to convey information and to interact with others and can also be used to explain solutions to problems verbally such as what to do when you are hungry or sleepy.

Five years: All basic sentence forms are usually intact by this age and there is an average length of utterance of five words. The language system is essentially that of adults although it may not be as complex and will not contain the same number of words in the vocabulary used.

It will be noted that in our discussion of language development, we have made no mention of a particular age at which certain "sounds" appear. Hall's (1962) and Healey's (1963) research has shown that there is no magical age at which a child acquires the /f/, the /b/, or any other sound. If you listen to the speech of young children, you will hear most sounds clearly articulated from a very early age by the majority of children. Reasons for misarticulations of certain sounds will be discussed in the chapter on articulation and related to specific developmental levels.

Summary

This chapter has been an overview of how our particular system of verbal communication develops. We have suggested that language develops both from innate programming and a feeling of utility within our society. Factors affecting these two concepts that have been discussed can be viewed from the section dealing with age-specific milestones discussed in Chapter II so that all areas can be integrated.

Chapter IV
ARTICULATION
ERRORS

Identification and Definition

Articulation refers to the way sounds are made, such as how the tongue and lips are positioned to form a particular individual sound, such as the /m/ or /p/. There is a general understanding among listeners of a given verbal communication system (language) that identifies whether a sound comes within what is considered normal limits or whether we sense something is wrong or misarticulated. This impression of misarticulation may be generally referred to as baby talk, lazy tongue movement, or any other of a variety of descriptive terms that imply the listener has some trouble understanding what's being said.

Individuals in the field of speech pathology have, of necessity, refined this identification process into a variety of articulation tests that may be administered to identify specifically what type and where problems occur. A list of most commonly used tests will be found in the reference section of this book (Goldman and Fristoe, 1969; McDonald, 1964; Templin and Darley, 1969). In general, tests consist of a specific set of words said by the individual being tested while the examiner listens for articulation of specific sounds contained within each word. For example, the /s/ sound may be evaluated within the word /soup/, /paste/, or /pass/. Sounds generally are categorized as (1) correctly articulated (spoken), (2) omitted, (3) distorted, or (4) substituted (another sound used in place of the one being tested). Thus, the following might be heard within the test situation:

(1) correct = soup
(2) omitted = _oup

(3) distorted = soup
(with the /s/ airstream coming out the sides of the mouth instead of in front)
(4) substitution = toup

There are several additional considerations that arise when discussing testing procedures. There are strong individual preferences among speech pathologists as to whether the tester should say the word first and then have the child repeat it (imitation method) or whether the response should initially be elicited from the child in answer to a question or naming of a specific test picture (elicited method). Each group feels their results are the most accurate, but research has shown that there have been little actual differences between the two methods.

Another variation that may occur within the test situation is the actual variability of correct and incorrect production of the same sound. Some of this variability may happen in response to different interactive factors with different examiners or may occur on one day and not another. An additional interesting fact may be the child's misarticulation of a sound at one place in a word but not in another. We will use the example of the /r/ sound. The correct and incorrect pronunciation of the same sound may occur in a test word (*railwoad*) or may occur in different words within a sentence (*R*ichard can *w*un).

It should be remembered that articulation testing is done on a phonetic basis, i.e., how the sounds are made and heard, not how they are written in words. For example, the initial sounds in these words would be phonetically the same but spelled differently, such as *c*ar and *k*ite or *c*elery and *s*un.

Incidence

There are varying reports as to actual incidence of speech and/or hearing problems in preschool or school-age populations. The following data can be found in Eisensen and Ogilvie (1971), as quoted from a report compiled by the United States Department of Health, Education, and Welfare regarding school age children.

PREVALENCE OF SPEECH DISORDERS IN SCHOOL AGE CHILDREN
(per 10,000 with each type of speech/hearing problem)

Type of Problem	Percent of Children with Problem	Number of Children with Problem per 10,000
Hearing		
Profound (deafness)	.12	12
Moderate	15-20	1,500-2,000
Distortion	not known	
Speech		
Articulation defects		
a. physiologic	4-6	400-600
b. organic		
cleft palate	1.5-2	150-200
cerebral palsy	1.3	130
Voice	10	1,000
Retarded Speech		
Development	5	500
Language disorders	no formula available	

The incidence of communication problems within a preschool-age population was published by the American Speech-Language-Hearing Association in 1978 (ASHA). This report was released by the Department of Health, Education, and Welfare and quoted a figure of 13 percent of Head Start children during the 1976-1977 school year being designated as handicapped. Approximately 50 percent of those with handicaps were speech impaired and 4 percent hearing impaired. The definition of "handicapped" as to speech is "identifiable disorders as receptive and/or expressive language impairment, stuttering, chronic voice disorders and serious articulation problems affecting social, emotional and/or educational achievement..." (Counts, 1981). This would probably then exclude children with articulation errors that were consistent but that did not significantly impair ability to communicate with the staff. These figures are somewhat at variance with the previously reported incidence, although it should be remembered that the two reports deal with different age group populations. However, a word should be said about the many discrepancies that can be found even among studies within the same age group. The most obvious reason is that uneven standards are applied to identification of a problem, i.e., is an articulation defect defined as presence of one sound substitution in the medial position of one tested word, or can it be defined as x number of sound substitutions beyond some arbitrarily set chronological age standard? In addition, an article by Evard and Sabers (1979) raised several questions as to test validity that should be considered when identifying a speech/language problem. Their article deals specifically with evaluating the speech and language skills of children from various ethnic-racial groups and the ways these populations relate to established norms. We are then left with an unanswered question as to actual incidence of specific speech difficulties unless sufficient information is included in a particular report with regard to criteria used, population studied, and inferences drawn from the statistics.

Speech disorders as viewed from the developmental speech aspect discussed in this book are all viewed as diagnostically significant. We believe that no speech problem occurs by happenstance, and each problem is the result of certain causal factors that must be dealt with if elimination of the difficulty is to occur in the most efficient and therapeutically helpful manner. Certain physiological exceptions are to be understood as outside the developmental concept. These may, but not necessarily will, include physical limitations such as might result from a cleft palate or hearing loss.

Causal versus Concurrent

The concept of causal versus concurrent factors should always be kept in mind when thinking about incidence of speech problems in certain populations. It is too easy to assume that a given physiological limitation will automatically result in a given speech problem. The human speech mechanism is capable of infinite adjustments to limitations. There are no certain sound substitutions, omissions, distortions, or language deficits that can automatically be associated with a specific neurological difficulty. Therefore, when assessing speech and language competency, it is important to separate out causal (those incidences in which a definite cause and effect relationship can be proven) from concurrent factors (those that occur at the same time but do not happen as a direct result of a given situation). For example, a child born with no usable hearing will be unable to develop language skills in the same way that a normally hearing child will be able to do. The lack of hearing is then a *causal* factor in speech and language difficulties. An example of *concurrent* factors might be the presence of both reading problems and articulation problems in the same third-grade boy. One difficulty does not necessarily automatically cause the other. The cause and effect relationship cannot be proven in this case.

Causal Factors

It is the premise of the developmental speech concept that sounds and voice quality carry an underlying meaning that we all unconsciously interpret and react to but are usually unaware of on the surface. There are many examples in everyday situations, even in the advertising field, that produce a reaction or interpretation on the part of the listener that means a certain message, either conscious or unconscious, has been sent by the speaker. A common example is the little child lisp adopted by grown-ups when wanting to portray the image of a young child, e.g., an actress doing an imitation of a little girl. For some reason, we are helped to complete the image of a young child by the presence of the lisp. The actress sends the message, and we receive it correctly as fitting into the character she wants us to imagine her being.

The advertising world has capitalized on this same set of underlying meaning of sounds by using a sound substitution for the /L/ in the word *little* when portraying the image of a young tiger wanting to get some additional closeness to his mother tiger during the eating of a particular brand of cereal. From some conscious or unconscious awareness, the advertising man who wrote that commercial knew that a certain sound and mothering/nurturance activities were all tied closely together and would be especially appealing to the young child watching television who would then press for the purchase of that particular brand of cereal.

These are only two of the many examples that can be found in everyday life if we are but tuned in to listen for them. The preceding two examples and others have been used many times in workshops that I have given, and I always receive the same responses from the audience about their interpretation of what different sounds are trying to portray. If we can then agree that these examples have meaning both to the sender and receiver of the misarticulated sound, we can then transfer this idea from the script of a play or the television screen to an application in real life. When discussing the misarticulations of young children, it must be remembered that they are not reading from a play script or from a television ad but are using the sounds that have meaning for certain general feelings or responses to relationships. McCarthy, as quoted in Byrne and Shervanian (1977), believes that "earliest sounds are intimately connected with physiological movements of breathing and sucking." Other sounds appear to be added to the sound repertoire as the introduction of more solid foods requires chewing. It seems plausible, then, to carry this idea further to suggest that sounds are associated not only with the physiological satisfaction or nonsatisfaction of bodily needs but also to the psychological issues that surround the satisfaction or nonsatisfaction of these needs. The idea of certain sounds being associated with specific developmental levels has been discussed in greater detail by Rousey (1982). However, for our current purposes the reader is asked to consider the general concept that sounds do have meaning, whether recognized or not, both to the speaker and to the listener that goes beyond the generally accepted use of communication by words.

Therefore, we are assuming that any child or adult who persists in maintaining a pattern of sound substitutions or distortions is doing so to satisfy and/or to try to notify significant people in the environment that there are certain developmental needs still remaining unmet. This idea could be termed the *red flag* concept, and it behooves those interested in the welfare of an individual with the speech problem to attend to this red flag and to recognize the problem and attempt to deal with it.

Specific Developmental Needs

Certain common developmental needs are particularly prevalent in the preschool years that must be met successfully in order to continue appropriate development later in life. These needs are especially important during the preschool years because during this time a child is forced either willingly or unwillingly to deal with many issues and has the opportunity successfully or unsuccessfully to meet these issues. These concepts have been discussed in some detail in Chapter II and will not be reviewed here except to relate them to specific behaviors or interactions within the context of a school/day care/home situation. By a proper speech screening technique and interpretation, these needs can be quickly and accurately identified. However, if this service is not available, another method that can be used is a critical analysis of behavior observed in a particular child that has incorrect patterns of speech. If the child has the behaviors described and speech errors, the caring adult should consider that a red flag has appeared and the child in question needs help. A critical analysis should include the following questions:

1. How would you describe the child's behavior when he first enters school, day care, or arrives home? For example, does the child always immediately need help taking off his coat or demand immediate attention from some significant adult in any situation? Behavior that would be a red flag would seem to go on for a longer period of time than seems necessary or could be seen in other children. The child in question might seem unable to get on with the business of the day without some special attention or recognition over and above appropriate levels.

2. Does the child ask for help when you know he is capable of doing an activity alone? This might take the form of needing help buttoning up a coat, tying shoes, or finding a particular toy that is in plain view. It would seem that the child is acting like and needing help on a much younger age level than you would expect from someone of his chronological age.

3. Does the child always seem to want to sit next to or on the lap of an available adult and seem to need a special amount of physical contact with others? It might seem that the child is often clinging to or needing a hug from adults.

4. Does this particular child always seem to be the last one to get ready to go out the door, prepare work or play materials, or generally be ready to participate in activities? There may be no overt observable delay, but somehow this one particular child never seems quite ready to participate as freely and easily

as other children in the group.

5. Does this child seem to withdraw rapidly from cooperation the harder you try to encourage or force participation? You may get the feeling that the harder you push him, the harder the child digs in his heels and refuses, often with more uncooperativeness or with silence.

6. Is this a child that seems particularly distrustful of what he can expect from adults? For example, he may not really believe that you will follow through on promises and will remember rightly or wrongly that you forgot a particular activity or promise and remind you of this error often.

7. Does this particular child consistently use bossy or ordering kinds of tough talk to get his way with others and always seem to be unable to use the words *please* and *thank you* or know appropriate ways of interaction with other children and adults?

8. Does the child quite often discuss the wonderful times or things at home, such as toys, activities, or food? He may also talk a lot about what he is missing by being at school or day care and seem to have thoughts of home quite often while away during the day.

9. Does the child seem to act too grown up and in charge of others to the degree that he spends too much time acting like a coteacher or coparent? Quite often this child will attempt to discipline or organize activities with the other children instead of feeling comfortable in his role as one of the children.

It is important to review these and associated questions with each speech-disordered child because children at this preschool age are usually still actively pursuing their particular needs and an appropriate behavioral analysis by a perceptive, caring adult will yield important information about specific developmental needs that remain unmet. All of the examples given previously will probably apply part of the time to most of the children you know, but it is important to analyze behavior that is consistent with one particular child over a period of time. The nine questions offered will give you an informal checklist to use in analyzing the behavior and give you a place to start doing a critical analysis. You may add other questions to this list that seem particularly important or relevant in a home, preschool, or day care setting. What is important is that you try to take an objective look at the behavior of a particular child in whom you are interested.

In addition to the somewhat more objective observations listed, there are some subjective judgments that should be included in this analysis. These subjective judgments can be rated individually and then compared to others who are involved in the care of the child in question. The first nine and the six additional judgments that follow can be put together to compose a comprehensive objective and subjective picture of a particular child, and then decisions can be made to more objectively plan for the needs and care of the child.

10. How does this child really make me feel? Some questions under this section might be: Am I happy when I see this child coming to school or coming home, or do I think the day will be easier for me and the other children if he is gone for a while? Does this child make me feel like a successful teacher or parent? Do I feel frustrated, happy, rejecting, motherly, or fatherly toward this child?

11. What would I do differently with this child? Would

I be more proud, stricter, reward more or less, punish more or less, or be more consistent with discipline or rules or praise?

12. What do I especially like about this child? Some qualities that easily come to mind are cheerfulness, good manners, special talents (such as art or music), and cleanliness. These and many others lend support to a good feeling between adults and children.

13. What do I especially dislike about this child? Some aspects that could be considered within this category are a negative attitude about people, a lack of warmth, and poor personal hygiene. These and other qualities contribute to a feeling of distance between adults and a particular child.

14. What kind of a home life or school experience do I think this child has? Would the parent or teacher be thought of as supportive or moderately or greatly interested in the child? Does the school or home environment seem unstable and chaotic or calm and consistent, and what effect does this have on the child? This question would, of course, be a rating of how the adult sees the opposite situation from the one they are directly involved with.

15. How do my attitudes about this child help or interfere with my job as his parent or teacher? This last question may involve some thoughtful analysis of an adult's behavior, and it may be helpful to discuss this last question with another person.

Admittedly, there are no quick and easy answers to either the first nine objective or the six following subjective questions, but if an honest attempt is made to answer each one of them, a fairly accurate picture can be drawn of a child and his relationship with adults. In the absence of a developmental speech analysis, this type of critical look by an interested, skillful, observant adult can provide invaluable insights into the developmental needs of a child that has given you a red flag signal of a speech problem. At this point, it may be important to rediscuss one of the popular misconceptions about speech problems that was discussed in Chapter I. You will remember that we stated that many adults believe that children will outgrow their speech problems and, therefore, nothing should be done except to wait. Those concerned with the basic underlying emotional and physical well-being of children know that it is far more advantageous and efficient to later development to meet a need while the child is still young before the problem expands or deepens. Early intervention is always more effective and quicker than later long-term work that may have let a child live with a problem over a period of several years.

It is not the purpose of this book to equate certain sound difficulties with certain developmental levels because the interpretation of test results needs the expertise of a professional familiar with the fields of speech pathology, child development, and audiology. However, if you are concerned about a particular child with some sounds that are mispronouced (misarticulated), you will find that the child will probably fit into a general behavior pattern or group of patterns that will coincide with the general developmental needs that we have discussed. The following sections will be divided into specific behavior description syndromes and particular activities that can be adapted to help the child meet his developmental need in the easiest possible way. If these needs are correctly identified and met, the particular misarticulation that prompted the initial critical analysis should disappear because the need for maintaining the misarticulation or causal factor will be eliminated. The child will then be free to grow, expand, and develop in the easiest possible manner. Remember, there are particular sound difficulties that will alert you to looking for these specific descriptions of behavior.

Admittedly, this method is not as efficient and precise as having an individual in the field of speech pathology who is also trained in child development and psychology who could pinpoint the particular areas of difficulty and then offer a specific plan to help alleviate the problem areas. However, if this service is not readily available, then the caring adult can be alerted to the needs of the child by looking at the behavior patterns described in following sections. Because it is sometimes difficult to obtain an objective measurement or description of the child when one does it alone, it might be helpful to use the How to See a Child checklist in the Appendix with one or more individuals who are concerned with the care of the child who would give a different perspective. This might be done with the parent and teacher working together or with a professional in one of the fields listed above.

We will list specific needs that are common to all preschool children and try to draw a comprehensive picture of how a child with this particular need might be described. Although people never fit neatly into a certain descriptive category, all of the information given within each of these sections should be taken as a general overall suggestion of things to look for or to be aware of in a particular child's behavior pattern. Again, you should be cautioned that the child may not always behave in exactly the same manner. It would be helpful to take several observational samples at different times of the day, different days of the week, in different situations, and with different adults. If this is done in a careful enough manner, you will see, if applicable, certain patterns that will begin to emerge and certain behavioral characteristics that seem to be fairly consistent. Again, if you are working in concert with another adult, it can be helpful to bring up even minor observations to have them confirmed or questioned by someone else.

Another point that needs to be emphasized is that all of the needs listed in the following section are ones that are not considered to be out of the ordinary but are well within the range of normal developmental situations that occur for all children. The point in question is that some children seem to need more than usual amounts of attention paid to certain areas. This need is quite often expressed through change or misarticulation in speech patterns and, therefore, is only alerting us to the fact that the child has not finished or felt sufficiently satisfied at one particular level in development. Therefore, the individual who can recognize and meet these needs will be doing a service to the child both in the present and in the future if this need can be met in the easiest and most efficient way possible. Children do not knowingly misarticulate sounds and are probably unaware of their misarticulation unless attention is paid to it by adults or other children. Therefore, misarticulations are springing from an internal need of the child, which he is attempting to play out through his misarticulations. The child does not deliberately set out to substitute a /w/ for /r/ sound to give a certain message. However, if you will remember in some of the earlier information presented in the book, the child has not mislearned the sound. Misarticulations are

made on an unconscious level by the child to express
needs in the same way that we can assess the behavior of a
child and know if he is sleepy or hungry by his actions.
We then can meet these needs by providing the appropriate remedy. Although we are presenting the following sections as *needs*, they are also indicative of specific sound
difficulties. However, we will not list the individual
sounds associated with each so that attention can be fo-
cussed on the broader behavior description.

Need for Successful Separation from Home

DESCRIPTION: A child who is having particular difficulty in successfully separating from home is one who
may spend a great deal of time talking about all the wonderful toys, food, people, etc., at home and imply that
school materials are second-rate. This child may also be
absent from school a great deal because of stomachaches,
headaches, or other nonspecific ailments. He always
seems to be in conflict over whether he wants to come to
school or would rather be at home. Although the child can
admit that school is good, home is also still better. A kin-
dergarten teacher told me that quite often children arrive
at school in September using the substitution associated
with this need, but by the middle of the year the misarticulation seems to have disappeared. Unknowingly she
was commenting on the growth of the children in her class
and their successful committment to coming to school after separating from home. The children who eliminated
this sound substitution were ones who were able to psychologically as well as physically leave their homes and
take part in the school experience. Quite often when I am
discussing this particular need many adults will say they
have the same kind of feeling, especially on Monday

mornings, when they wish they could stay at home but know that they have to go ahead and go to work on time. This would also be true of people who have had to move from one section of the world to another but whose heart remains in their original homeland. There is also the feeling of one foot being in the new country and one foot being back in the homeland. Adults are able to verbalize these feelings on a more abstract level and to take certain measures that will make us feel better about separating from one situation and going to another. Therefore we do not need to rely on sound substitutions to express our feelings but can use words and talk about our problems with separation.

The conflict that many children feel is illustrated by a little boy who said that he liked school okay but every day when he got home from school and wanted some orange juice to drink, his little sister had drunk it all up while he was gone and left none for him. In other words, he equated this with all the good things being usurped by his sister, and nothing good that happened at school could compare with the disappointment he felt upon arriving home. In addition, you can imagine that the thought of his sister and mother sitting at home together drinking the juice must have crossed his mind several times a day while he was at school. Another example is the little girl who told me with great sorrow that her mother always made her come to school whether she wanted to or not, while her older brother got to stay at home whenever he wanted. Whether the actual veracity of these incidents is accurate or not, what is important is the feeling that the child was experiencing and causing the conflict over home separation.

PRESCRIPTION: The main emphasis on helping a child

through home separation difficulties is to *sell* the idea that being away from home and experiencing new activities and situations is a desirable thing. This is not to downplay feelings of home being a good place but only to emphasize that other places can also be good places to be. Some specific suggestions are the following:

1. Replaying through the actual experience of getting ready to come to school/day care, i.e., getting dressed, riding in the car, the moment of separation from home and/or parent, the home-going time, and discussing the feelings that the child associates with each event.

2. Talking about or drawing pictures of differences and similarities of school and home, emphasizing the good and not so good points of each. For instance, you might say that at school and at home there are grown-ups who take care of you, read you stories, give you things to eat, and play with you. However, at school there are special friends and a different variety of books and toys that are always available.

3. Positive talk about the advantages of being old enough to leave home and to be able to come to school. You might talk about a younger sibling being left at home who does not get to go on field trips to the zoo, get the special snacks you always have, or have the chance to play on all the climbing equipment.

4. Emphasize the predictable routine of school and availability of teachers, toys, food, and other children. Each day there are new things to do and learn, all within the context of a regular schedule that the child is familiar with.

5. Before leaving school at the end of the day, the

teacher might discuss the next day's activities so that the child is able to look forward to specific plans. This gives the child a chance to know that a particular event is going to take place the next day and he will have a certain special reason to want to come back the next day.

6. If a child is wanting to bring a toy from home, he is probably having some difficulty in separation and is bringing a piece of security with him so that in times of stress he can rely on this subject for reassurance. It is important to talk with the child about this so that he understands that objects can be lost or broken but the thoughts and feelings from home can be carried within him. The feelings are the same when a child is trying to take home a toy or other article from school. It is a sign that he needs a piece of the good environment to carry with him. A good way to handle this is to help substitute a hug for the object and to tell the child that he can never lose the good feeling in his mind about how the hug felt with your arms around him. ·

7. It is important to be aware of any part that adults may be playing in difficulty with home separation. This is an excellent opportunity for parent-teacher discussion about the role of school and home in the child's life and the positive effects each can have, but in different ways. Because of particular family relationships, sometimes it is difficult for a parent to feel completely free about sending a youngster off to the school or day care and the child will sense this indecision about separation and probably feel the same indecision and not feel good about leaving. There should be a calm assurance on the part of parents

that they know their child will be perfectly safe and have a good time away and that they are glad the child is able to go. Parents may need to tell the child that they would not have him in a situation where they did not feel there would be good care. It is also important that parents and teachers work out differences of opinion with regard to discipline and general child care so that the child does not feel any conflict of loyalty between home and school. It may be that some things need to be openly discussed concerning different types of behavior at home or school. Simply because the situation and people are different does not mean that one is better than the other. It just means that the child will be expected to have a good time and be well cared for in all situations.

Parenting/Nurturance Need

DESCRIPTION: A child who still has mothering needs will be one who works very hard to sit next to the teacher or on the teacher's lap during story time, field trips, etc., and who enjoys any type of physical closeness. There is a general communication of needing to be taken care of. A teacher may voice the feeling that the child clings continuously and that she cannot get away from this closeness. Also, this child may spend a good deal of time in the housekeeping area busily engaged in mothering/fathering the dolls in an attempt to play through the developmental need he feels. A word of caution should be inserted regarding the *quality* of nurturance a child is receiving. In one instance the mother of a child still needing help in the parenting/nurturance area was very active in public areas of child care, i.e., driving on field trips, but the teacher of the little girl made the comment that there was a definite feeling of distance between the mother and child. There was no feeling of warmth or nurturance going from mother to child despite the pose of the devoted mother.

PRESCRIPTION: A general feeling of physical and emotional closeness should be stressed with the child in need of nurturance. An emphasis should be put on doing *for* and giving *to* in daily activities. Some specific suggestions might be as follows:

1. Sit next to these children at snack or mealtimes and talk about the good feeling the activity gives everyone.
2. Arrange for lots of physical closeness and verbally recognize the feeling of warmth that emanates from this closeness.
3. Spend time with the child in housekeeping activities. This could be cooking for the child and feeding and then talking about the experience. This adds emphasis to the parenting or nurturance idea that appeals to many children. It may also be important for the child to take the role of the parent and experience the feeling of taking care of and feeding other people.
4. The adult should emphasize appropriate feelings of *giving* freely to the child. This giving could be in the form of help in general activities, not just in tangible objects. It should be emphasized that the adult is there to give as much help as is needed until the child is able to do things on his own comfortably.
5. The child should be helped to know that the feeling of closeness can last in his mind all day. Thus, a parent or teacher can make the child feel loved and cared for even though they are apart. You can also

talk with the child about feeling lonesome for a parent during the day but at the same time helping him remember some special thing about the parent that will help him know that he is loved, such as the hug the parent gave him earlier in the day. This can also be done with regard to the warm feelings that are engendered at the school during the day that can last until the return to school the next day.

Need for Trusting

DESCRIPTION: In order for a child to freely interact with others there must be a basic trust in people and the world. A typical remark of a child with this particular difficulty was concerned with the fact that his mother promised many times over to buy him some new toys and to bring them when she returned from work. However, the boy sadly acknowledged that his mother never kept her promise. This is a child that wants to believe what adults tell him and continues to hope but is never sure that any promise will be fulfilled. Therefore the basic trust that this boy is trying to develop continues to be thwarted in its development and makes it difficult for the boy to believe other promises that are made to him. The reality of the situation is that the mother is probably unaware of the mistrust she continues to foster and is only using her promise of toys to alleviate whatever feelings she and her son may have that revolve around the leave-taking situation. However, continued disappointment leads to distrust of others and a forced, unnatural dependence on self-gratification. There is an overly developed interest and concentration on the *self* and its well-being.

PRESCRIPTION: These children need to develop a trust toward and dependence on others in their environment that can be relied upon in a continuing manner. A teacher, parent, or caretaker can foster a feeling of acceptance of the child that is dependable and constant. This can be done through a consistent reliability of actions and words. Specific suggestions might be the following:

1. Verbalizing the idea that when promises are made, promises are kept. For example, if a trip to the zoo is planned for the next day, a reminder on the day of the trip that the promise was being kept is an important way of fostering this sense of trust and reliability. If occasional disappointments must occur, they can be viewed within the larger context of general reliability and promises kept.

2. Telling the child that he knows you are always glad to see him on arrival at school or home and that you will always greet him by name and with a welcoming word. Even if the morning has started badly and the child arrives at school in tears, you will still be there to greet him and be glad to see him. Thus the idea is fostered that the adult is dependable and reliable no matter what the fluctuating state of moods the child may be experiencing. The relationship is solid and can be counted on, no matter what the environmental circumstances may be.

3. Providing a somewhat set routine for daily activities so that a child can learn what to expect. This routine, of course, has to be set within normal flexibility of the day's activities. When a child learns that there is a fixed orderly feeling to his day, then he can trust the environment and be sure what is expected of him within this environment.

4. The most important thing is that the child knows that there are certain important adults in his life

that he can depend on for love and care. In a larger sense, this is an important need for all humans. If we can know that we have a dependable reliable base in our lives, then we can be free to expand our horizons and explore new activities with safety because the solid base is always there to rely on when we feel the need.

Need for Age-appropriate Behavior

DESCRIPTION: On the surface a child with this sound substitution may appear to be very grown-up and responsible. One particular child that comes to mind is one who spent a great deal of time being the boss of activities in the classroom and would report infractions of all rules that he happened to observe. In a sense he was setting himself up as the other adult in the classroom and felt in charge of the other children. Sometimes children will, rightly or wrongly, feel they have been put in charge of younger brothers and sisters and are unhappy about having to assume the role of a care taking adult while they are still in the process of needing to be taken care of themselves. Another example is that of an eight-year-old girl in the third grade who, during the therapy time, insisted on sitting in kindergarten-size chairs because it felt so good to sit in a little girl chair. She was able almost immediately to launch into a description of the large number of adult responsibilities she felt she was forced to assume at home concerned with taking care of a younger brother. She admitted she secretly enjoyed crawling into the baby bed and pretending she was the youngest one in the family. These vignettes sum up the feelings of a child who has not satisfactorily had his/her infantile needs met to a sufficient degree to enable them to continue to grow and fully participate in the feelings and activities expected in age-appropriate behavior. A common phrase these children quite often hear is, "You are a big girl/boy," which is exactly what they do not want to be yet.

PRESCRIPTION: Children in this type of behavior pattern need to be encouraged to be as young as they feel the need to be in order for them to finish up the work of being young or a little child. The following are some specific suggestions.

1. All demands for grown-up behavior should be eliminated along with remarks that suggest that they should act grown-up or act their age. What a child is trying to say is that he or she does not feel comfortable with the expectations adults have placed on them for this more mature behavior. Quite often this problem can be found in children who are unusually big or tall for their age. Somehow a four-year-old who has the physical look or size of a five- or six-year-old will be expected to act like a five- or six-year-old instead of the four-year-old, which puts an unnatural level of behavior expectation on the child.

2. Be aware of the role that adults play in encouraging this type of behavior because this child is usually very helpful to have around the home or class. They do not require constant help and can often assume the role of taking care of other children.

3. Do role-playing activities and discuss how it might feel to be the youngest one in the family and how they would act. For example, you might talk about how younger children in the family would need help getting dressed or playing with toys.

4. Special attention needs to be given to let this type of child know that he is not in charge of the classroom

or home. Continual reminders may need to be given that there is only one adult who is completely in charge and is the only one who gives directions and orders. All children in the situation are just that, *children*, and do not need to assume any of the responsibility for management.

5. In families it is important that children not be put in charge of younger siblings when they are not ready for this type of responsibility. There is a difference between being in charge of younger siblings and helping the parents in a shared responsibility. The child needs to know that there is always a responsible adult who has the ultimate authority for caretaking, and anything they do is only being done under the direction of the appropriate adult.

Need for Cooperation, Sharing, Participation

DESCRIPTION: A child who has difficulty in these particular areas is characterized quite often as stubborn, strong willed, sneaky, or resistive. A good example of a child in this category is a little girl who was in a classroom that was being screened for speech problems. The teacher described her as on the surface being very sweet and cooperative but agreed that her behavior during the screening carried over into many school activities. The entire class had been screened except for one last person according to the number of enrolled pupils. The discrepancy and missing child was discussed audibly by the teacher and examiner and the teacher asked the class who had not been out in the hall to say the words with the examiner. When no answer was forthcoming, there was a check of names on the roster. The result was that the one missing child was sitting in a chair directly below where the teacher and examiner were standing and yet an effective resistance had been mounted by this girl by simply silently sitting. When her omission was discovered, she came willingly and sweetly, but she had still effectively controlled the situation by her actions.

This type of controlling or manipulative behavior is usually done without any overt sign of resistive action. Control can be exercised by just *not doing*, i.e., always managing to be the one that holds up the recess line because a glove is lost or is the last one to finish up a work project because of dropped pencils, etc. The more cooperation is insisted upon, the harder the child will seem to dig in his/her heels, and ways not to cooperate will be strengthened. A child in this category is struggling with the general developmental level discussed in Chapter II of learning to conform or to defy adult wishes. Conforming or cooperating is difficult to do, and yet the child does not have the verbal means to express this resistance; therefore, it takes the form of physical defiance or noncooperation.

PRESCRIPTION: This type of child needs to feel that he has some voice in his own decision making in terms of cooperation because he has not yet learned to conform (cooperate) to acceptable standards of behavior without a form of defiance.

1. Cooperation will be more easily achieved if the child feels that he has a choice to make in terms of behavior. This choice must be offered within the framework or structure of acceptable standards. *Examples*: When a child does not want to sit down with the class, he can be offered the choice of sitting in one chair *or* another so that the child conforms to adult request, but still has a choice in the matter.

The adult should not present the request as —

(a) Do you want to sit down or not? (which could result in one unacceptable behavior choice for the adult), or

(b) I will force you to sit down (which results in an unacceptable behavior choice only for the child), or

(c) I don't care whether you sit down or not (which results in an unacceptable choice for only the adult).

2. When certain cooperation must be insisted upon, such as staying with a group while crossing the street, the choice can be given in words to the effect, "You can either do it yourself, or I will help you do it." This allows the child to make a choice and if the adult needs to apply discipline, it can be done by holding the child's hand during street crossing while verbalizing the fact that it was the child's choice that he needed to have the adult help him cross the street instead of choosing to do it by himself. It is hoped that the child will be able to internalize these structured limits of behavior and learn that the acceptable choice is for him to learn to apply limits himself instead of always needing someone else to do it for him.

3. The reason behind all this silent passive-aggressive technique is the child's inability to openly express defiance and anger verbally instead of in actions. Therefore it is important to help the child learn to express his anger in appropriate verbal ways that will enable him to handle his feelings in a more socially acceptable manner. This can be done by teachers, parents, and other adults appropriately expressing displeasure themselves so that a role model is provided.

4. It is important for the child to know that expressing anger will in no way endanger the relationship he has with others. He can learn that it is a safe thing to do and his anger can be accepted by others without being returned in kind.

Need for Self-concept/Identity

DESCRIPTION: Children with undeveloped self-concepts seem to be unsure of themselves and reluctant to assert themselves appropriately in terms of their needs and wants. There is a lack of self-assurance about their activities, both verbally and physically. In addition, there most probably will be some undeveloped sense of their identity as a boy or girl. They will be unsure of how a grown-up girl would act as a lady or a grown-up boy act as a man. There may be some crossing over or a blurring of these roles because they have not had appropriate adult role models with which to identify. It is important for children to have both male and female adults with which to compare or contrast their own perceptions of being a boy or girl. Sometimes the living arrangements do not provide readily available male and female adults, and it is important for parents and teachers to try to make up for this, either through visitors in the home or school or appropriate relatives. Specific suggestions might be as follows:

1. Discussion and description of adult male and female models, i.e., how men and women differ in terms of voices, body size, physical movement, activities, and clothing. They can pretend to be a dad or mom in the morning and talk about how dad acts while shaving or mother looks while putting on make up, etc.

2. Discussion of the children's own physical characteristics, such as size and color of hair and can also include special creative talents or things that are enjoyed such as singing, drawing, climbing trees, or talking with people.
3. Appropriate expressions of self-assertiveness should be encouraged, such as feeling that he has equal rights and privileges within the class or family setting and can expect that these rights will be honored by everyone.
4. Adults should emphasize the idea that there are special differences between males and females and that these differences do not imply value judgments as to self-worth or preconceived ideas as to specific roles in life that either sex will be expected to follow. The important point here is that there are differences, but these are based on certain inherent characteristics that are part of being a boy or girl and allow each of us to play a particularly important role with others.

Need for Appropriate Verbal Assertiveness

DESCRIPTION: A child with this particular sound substitution finds it very difficult to verbalize needs appropriately. The role of a tough guy seems to be the method the child assumes in verbal interaction with others. There is a preponderance of bossy, ordering, tough talk when playing with other children and talking with adults. Requests are not cushioned with a semblance of politeness or social phrases such as, "Please give me the ball." Rather, the situation would demand from this child a simple "Gimme" with an accompanying physical action.

PRESCRIPTION: Limits need to be set for verbal expression and physical expression of rights. Here are some suggestions.

1. An active discussion by adults should be provided that explores the differences between appropriate and tough ways to interact verbally in a variety of situations, such as during play, meal times, or group activities.

2. The teacher or parent might have such a discussion with a small group of children and have them assume various roles while practicing asking for turns, second helpings at meals, or permission to enter a group activity. This would include standing up for themselves in disagreements and being able to settle things through verbal, amicable means.

3. An important role for the teacher or parent is to provide models for children to observe in their verbal interactions with others. It is important for children to hear adults using appropriate ways of verbal interaction such as asking people to do certain things and then remembering to thank them afterward. This would also include adults standing up for their own rights with others. All these interactions should be done in a natural manner by adults so that they seem part of the daily routine.

4. It is important to include recognition of when children do use appropriate means of verbal interaction with others. After a child has asked for a turn with a toy or has been able to say that they prefer doing one thing over another, the adult would be advised to recognize the good way of using language so that the child receives some positive feedback for his efforts.

Summary

A general summary of children with various behavior characteristics that correlate with specific speech (articulation) difficulties has been presented. No attempt to relate specific sounds with specific behavior patterns has been made. This has been done deliberately so that no cookbook method of dealing with children or their sound substitutions will be possible. It cannot be emphasized too much that each child is unique and that it is the behavior and underlying need on a developmental level that needs to be dealt with for an effective speech therapy to occur. Therefore, it is the responsibility of the reader to think about each child about whom there are concerns and to determine which of the preceding behavior syndromes seem to fit him best and to act accordingly.

Chapter V
STUTTERING
(DISFLUENCY)

Identification

There are a number of definitions of what constitutes stuttering behavior, but for purposes of our book, we will use a commonly accepted description of an abnormal number of disfluences which consist of hesitations, blocks, repetition of syllables, sounds or words, and/or prolongations. The key word in this definition is *abnormal* because any speaker has some disfluency in speech. We all range along the continuum from fluent to disfluent according to circumstances, our physical and emotional health, degree of pressure, and other factors. There is a difference also that should be noted between stuttering and cluttering. The latter is usually defined as consisting of a torrent of words, poorly or partially articulated so that the listener has the impression of jumbled speech. However, if a clutterer is asked to slow down, there will be an immediate improvement in speech production and in the smoothness of speech flow. This may or may not happen with a person who stutters.

It has been estimated that 85 percent of people

diagnosed as stutterers started before the age of five and the other 15 percent before seven years of age. The problem occurs in approximately 1 percent of the population in all cultures. The great majority of those who reported being former stutters felt they had a complete recovery of fluent speech. Statistical studies have indicated that stuttering occurs more frequently in boys than girls, at a ratio of 4:1 (Wingate, 1978). An interesting but unexplained phenomenon is that even severe stutterers will experience little difficulty when singing or speaking in unison. There often also seems to be a reduction in stuttering behavior when the individual is talking to younger children or talking aloud with no listener present. Speech will also be easier when the same material is read or spoken aloud repeatedly over a concentrated period of time.

Causation

Literally hundreds of research studies have been conducted to determine the cause of stuttering behavior that could then lead to a specific cure or remedy. So far the most that these studies have been able to document is in the area of what does not cause stuttering. There have been no consistent findings in the areas of personality disorder, physiological differences, the influence of intelligence, heredity, or specific environmental interactions. The question still remains whether there is one yet undetermined cause or whether there is multiple causation. Therefore, our view of the problem deals with description of behavior and particular therapeutic measures that have been proven to be effective in the treatment of individuals who stutter. This is not to say that there are not strong believers in various theories, because a number of people have hypothesized a particular causation and developed a very specific effective set of therapy techniques stemming from their theory.

This book will review in general terms several of the major theories as to causation of stuttering, keeping in mind that there is no universally accepted cause or etiology of the problem. One theory that has been investigated is that children who stutter and who continue to do so have a constitutional predisposition inherited in their neurophysiological makeup. This predisposition is then triggered by events or conditions in the environment. A second theory is that there is a misevaluation by adults of a child's normal nonfluencies, which then escalates the speech behavior into a problem because of the anxiety and frustration projected onto the child. Others have advanced the idea that stuttering is somehow linked to a manifestation of a personality or psychological problem in the self-concept. Others have suggested that the exact cause is not so important as what seems to maintain, support, or reward the stuttering behavior. It can be determined from this overview that there is a wide divergence of opinion concerned with etiology, ranging from physical to emotional or a combination of both. Regardless of the theory, most experts are in agreement as to what should be done to alleviate any difficulty with speech in the preschool child.

In attempts to trace the course of stuttering from the first fairly easy repetitions to the almost totally disabling blockage of speech, researchers have tried to define stages that will accurately plot the progress of the difficulty in hopes of finding some clue as to what causes the problem to either disappear or progress. It has been suggested that even the first easy repetitions of true stutterers are somehow different than those of the individual whose problem goes away after a brief period. However, no objective system has been devised to differentiate the true from the temporary stutterer so far. Part of the difficulty is that so many of the attitudes associated with stuttering are hard to measure quantitatively. These include such subjective topics as frustration, anxiety, or embarrassment. It is important to remember when discussing stuttering and related observations that there are three main categories of reactions: (1) overt manifestation that can be objectively measured by observation, which includes such things as number of sounds or words repeated in a sentence or the time length of sound prolongations, (2) covert measurements, such as heart rate changes during stuttering, and (3) inferred changes such as anxiety connected with the stuttering. Every attempt should be made to define the type of reaction being discussed accurately, as well as the way it was obtained.

Stages/Phases of Stuttering

Although it is assumed that most preschool children will be included in the first, or primary, stages of stuttering behaviors, the continuum of the whole spectrum will be presented to give an overall view of the problem. A review of the literature (Bloodstein, 1969; Van Riper, 1971; Williams, 1971) indicates that stuttering behavior can roughly be divided into four general stages/phases or levels.

Level One: Any stuttering behavior only occurs infrequently and often is most apparent when there is an attempt to communicate verbally during periods of great excitement. There is very little awareness or concern about any difficulty.

Repetition of whole words, single sounds, or syllables will be the most frequent.

Level Two: There is still very little concern or anxiety, but stuttering behavior is more chronic, and the individual may begin to think of himself as a stutterer. The repetitions may turn into prolongations, and there may be some hesitancy associated with speaking.

Level Three: There is an increased awareness of speech difficulty on the part of the speaker and a definite feeling of frustration. The repetitions may become forced as the speaker tries to push the words/sounds out, and an individual may start to use tricks such as finger snapping to help him through difficult situations.

Level Four: There are now specific feared words/sounds, and the speaker makes determined efforts to avoid speaking situations where he anticipates difficulty.

Of course there is some overlapping between stages, and there may be additional clues that help to identify the level of stuttering, but in general this list should help the interested adult pinpoint the particular level at which stuttering is manifesting itself.

Parent/Teacher Dos and Don'ts

There are certain dos and don'ts that are commonly given to adults who are concerned about the child in the first level or primary stage of stuttering. These include the following suggestions.

DOS

1. Make speaking as pleasant as possible and facilitate the easy flow of speech with such activities as singing, reading, and talking in unison. These methods reduce the amount of pressure on a young child for speech production because usually words are familiar and are often used over and over. Also, it is uncommon for anyone to stutter when singing or speaking in unison. Hence, a child will know that there are times when speech is very easy and he can feel positive about the talking experience.

2. Help the child to handle easily any disruptive factors, such as other people trying to interrupt the conversation. This may involve the adult helping the child at first by saying, "Bobby wants to talk right now; please don't interrupt. You can have a turn later." It is important for a child to know that he has a right to his own period of conversation time and that this right cannot be easily overrun by other children or adults.

3. Eliminate any competing environmental stimuli, such as talking while the television is going, while the radio is playing, or when there seems to be a great deal of confusion in the vicinity of the child. All of these things tend to distract the child from speaking because he is trying to listen to other things that are going on as well as talk at the same time.

4. Alter any environmental pressures that seem to produce a negative reaction, such as time pressure. This may involve adults eliminating from their

conversation such words as "Hurry up," or "I'm tired of waiting for you," or any other expressions that seem to produce a feeling of impatience or pressure with regard to the child's attempts to talk.

5. Analyze situations that seem to produce more stuttering. Look at what the child is talking about or to whom, the time of day, and the reactions of others. It may be important to keep a daily log, without making a big production of it, so that you can get some kind of an idea if there is a pattern as to when the suttering seems to occur most frequently.

6. Analyze situations that seem to produce less or no stuttering in the same way so that you have a picture of when speech seems to be the easiest. You can then compare the information and, one would hope, get a picture of the child's general speech patterns, with regard to stuttering.

7. Listen carefully. Be the kind of listener that gives full attention and interest to the speaker. Quite often adults may be trying to read the newspaper, watch television, cook dinner, pay bills, or do a myriad of other activities while a child is trying to relate something that seems very important to him. The child is quite naturally distressed over this half attention and feels in competition with whatever activities seem to have equal or more importance than him.

8. Make speech activities and expectations age appropriate and realistic. Be aware of the type of language that can be expected from preschool children and do not put unrealistic pressure on a child to produce language that is more complex than should be expected from a preschooler.

9. Look at the relationship between the child and

important people in his world. Does it seem to be for the most part a good relationship that produces the kind of environment that allows the child to grow and expand his world at his own pace? Some of the questions that were discussed in Chapter IV would be important to review at this point and may give some additional information about the relationships that exist between the child and parent and/or the child and other caretakers.

DON'TS

1. Call attention to the child's difficult way of talking or refer to it as trouble. This gives a negative feeling to the child's attempts at communication, which may affect more than just the times of disfluency and may make him feel that all of his speech attempts are troublesome or difficult. In reality, usually a child in the primary stage of stuttering has many more periods of fluency than disfluency, and it is important to let him feel that, for the most part, he has an easy way of talking.

2. Use the word *stutterer* in the first or primary stages. The reason is because the word stutterer has an unknown connotation to the child and makes him feel that he has become something for which he has no reference. If you are discussing the child's speech, it would be better to more realistically describe what happens, such as "Sometimes you just say a word two or three times before you go on to the next one." This is an objective description of what happens and allows the child to know exactly what you are talking about.

3. Tell the child to slow up, repeat himself, or take a deep breath. These types of instructions usually

serve only to increase the pressure on the child for clear speech. If some of the other suggestions under the *Dos* section are implemented, the child will naturally slow up, be more relaxed, and not feel in such a hurry to speak.

4. Become impatient with the child's efforts at talking. Again, this only increases the child's anxiety about talking and probably will increase the number of disfluencies that are present. The important thing is for the child to know you have the time and interest in listening to him. Realistically, there are times when you do not have the time to listen. An adult may be having a conversation with another adult or child or be involved in an activity that must be continued or finished. It is important to say to the child, "I cannot listen to you right now with all of my attention because I must finish this project. However, I do want to hear what you have to say and when I have finished, I will sit down with you and give you all my attention, and I will remember that you wanted to talk with me." Thus, the idea is communicated that the adult is not under pressure to stop but still wants to know what the child has to say.

5. Ask the child to talk in high risk situations, such as when he is tired, in a hurry, or angry. It may be important for the adult to recognize these feelings for the child and say words to the effect, "I know it is difficult for you to tell me how angry you were when somebody hit you. It will be easier for you to tell me when you are not so upset."

6. Demand answers from the child that involve questions that are difficult or impossible to answer, such

as "Why did you cut your finger?" or "Why did you spill your juice?" These questions obviously would be hard for anyone to answer and increase the pressure on speaking.

Therapy for Older Children

Once the individual's speech patterns have passed from the first, or primary, level of stuttering, it is usually dealt with in a more direct, open manner. There is a combination of altering environmental pressures and direct work and discussion with the person concerning his stuttering. Specific practice techniques may be incorporated into the person's speech patterns such as learning to bounce, glide, or ease into initiating word production. There will also be more direct work on the feelings and attitudes of the person who stutters about speech and what he can do himself to monitor or change his feelings and self-image, if need be. Once beyond the first level of stuttering, therapy is usually directed by a speech pathologist in cooperation with the parents.

When to Refer to a Speech Pathologist

Although there is no general rule to follow concerning the exact time to seek the help of a professional speech pathologist, the following can be used as guidelines.

1. When the repetitions or other behaviors persist longer than six months, seek help.
2. When there seems to be a degree of frustration or anxiety during speaking situations that result in increased verbal difficulty, seek help.
3. When the child seems to avoid speaking situations because of decreased confidence in fluent speaking ability, seek help.

Remember any child may go through a period of normal word/sound repetitions and outgrow this habit with no undue attention or treatment. It is only when the problem persists or becomes a problem for the child or parent that professional help should be consulted. A first step might be to contact the child's pediatrician for guidance on when and to whom a possible referral might be made.

APPENDIX

How To See A Child

1. What is the child's behavior when first arriving at or leaving school or when leaving or coming home?

   <u>Takes care of needs</u>   <u>Sometimes needs attention/help</u>   <u>Always needs extra help/attention</u>

Comments:

2. How does the child react to discipline?

   <u>Responds easily</u>   <u>Needs reminding of rules, etc.</u>   <u>Rejects discipline, openly or silently</u>

Comments:

3. How does the child participate in activities?

   <u>Cooperates</u>   <u>Needs encouragement</u>   <u>Refuses on any terms</u>

Comments:

4. How would I describe this child?

Happy   Acts age appropriate   Preoccupied

Sad   Distrustful   Eager

Grown-up   Acts younger than age   Stubborn

Cooperative   Others

Comments:

5. How does this child make me feel?

Successful   Frustrated   Parental

Happy   Sad   Other

Comments:

6. What do I especially like about this child?

Behavior   Appearance   Special skills

Attitude   Other

Comments:

7. What is difficult about this child?

Behavior   Appearance   Attitude   Other

Comments:

8. How do I view this child's future?

   <u>Successful</u> ·<u>Difficult</u>   <u>Unknown</u>

Comments: (i.e. areas of special concern)

9. How would I most like to help this child?

   <u>Educational</u>   <u>Social skills</u>   <u>Physical skills</u>   <u>Other</u>

Comments:

REFERENCES

ASHA, 6.5% of Head Start Children are Speech Impaired, says HEW, June 1978, Vol. 20, 495.

Bloodstein, Oliver, *A Handbook on Stuttering*, National Easter Seal Society for Crippled Children and Adults. Chicago, Ill., 1969.

Byrne, Margaret C. and Shervanian, Chris C., *Introduction to Communicative Disorders*. New York: Harper and Row, 1977.

Counts, Theresa, Director, Topeka, U.S.D. #501 Head Start Program. Personal Communication from National Head Start Office regarding definition of speech handicap, 1981.

Doll, Edgar, *Vineland Social Maturity Scale*. Circle Pines, Minn., American Guidance Service, Inc., 1965.

Eisenson, Jon and Olgivie, Mardel, *Speech Correction in the Schools*. New York: MacMillan Publishing Co., Inc., 1971.

Engel, George, *Psychological Development in Health and Disease*. Philadelphia: W.B. Saunders Co., 1963.

Evard, Beth and Sabers, Darrell, "Speech and Language Testing with Distinct Ethnic-Racial Groups: A Survey of Procedures for Improving Test Validity." *Journal of Speech and Hearing Disorders*, 1979, *44*, 271-281.

Fraiberg, Selma, *The Magic Years*. New York: Charles Scribner's Sons, 1959.

Frankenburg, William E. and Dodds, Josiah, *Denver Developmental Screening Test*. University of Colorado Medical Center, 1969.

Goldman, R. and Fristoe, M., *Goldman-Fristoe Test of Articulation*. Circle Pines, Minn.: American Guidance Service, Inc., 1969.

Hall, W.F., A Study of the Articulation Skills of Children from Three to Six Years of Age. Unpublished doctoral dissertation, University of Missouri, 1962.

Healey, W.C., A Study of the Articulatory Skills of Children from Six to Nine Years of Age. Unpublished doctoral dissertation, University of Missouri, 1963.

Knobloch, Hilda and Pasamanick, Benjamin, *Gessel and Amatruda's Developmental Diagnosis*. New York: Harper and Row, 1974.

Lenneberg, Eric, *Biological Foundations of Language*. New York: John Wiley and Sons, Inc., 1967.

McDonald, E.T., *A Deep Test of Articulation*. Pittsburgh: Stanwix House, 1964.

Rousey, Carol, and Rousey, Clyde, L., *Your Child's Speech and Hearing*. Private publication, (booklet), 1978.

Rousey, Clyde L., "Techniques of Therapy Based on Principles of Psycho-Therapy." In *Current Therapy of Communication Disorders*, edited by William H. Perkins. New York: Thieme-Stratton, Inc., 61-71, 1982.

Templin, M.C. and Darley, F.L., *The Templin-Darley Test of Articulation*, 2nd ed. Iowa City: Bureau of Educational Research and Service, Division of Extension and University Services, University of Iowa, 1969.

Van Riper, Charles, *The Nature of Stuttering*. Englewood Cliffs, N.J.: Prentice-Hall, Inc., 1971.

Williams, Dean, "Stuttering Therapy for Children." In *Handbook of Speech Pathology and Audiology*, edited by Lee Travis. New York: Appleton Century Crofts, 1073-1093, 1971.

Wingate, Marcel, "Disorders of Fluency." *In Speech, Language and Hearing*, edited by Paul Skinner and Ralph Shelton. Reading, Mass: Addison-Wesley Publishing Co., 245-271, 1978.

Zimmerman, Irla Lee, Steiner, Violette, and Evatt, Roberta, *Preschool Language Scale*. Columbus, Ohio: Charles E. Merrill, 1969.

INDEX